YOUR KNOWLEDGE HAS VALUE

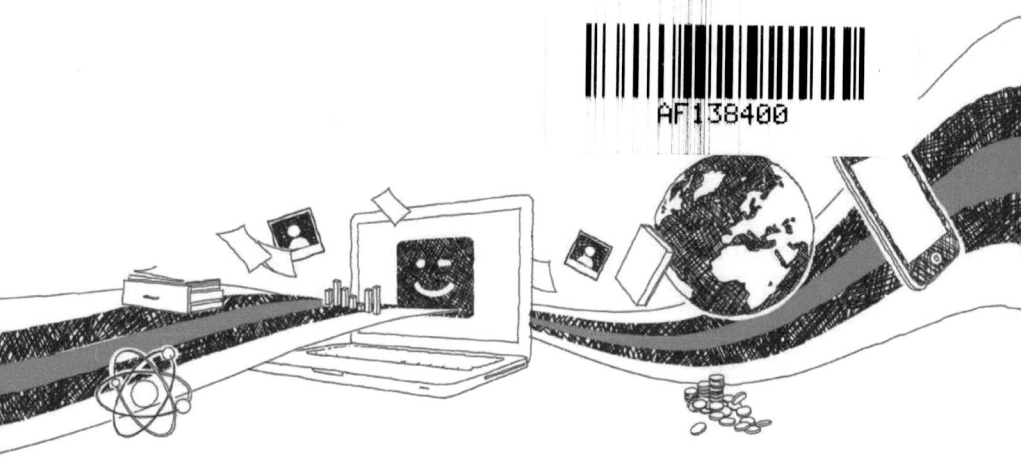

AF138400

- We will publish your bachelor's and master's thesis, essays and papers

- Your own eBook and book - sold worldwide in all relevant shops

- Earn money with each sale

Upload your text at www.GRIN.com
and publish for free

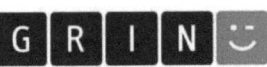

The Efficacy Of Herbal Mixtures On Some Bacteria. Staphylococcus aureus and Streptococcus pyogene

Bamidele Ijigbade

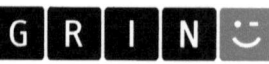

Bibliographic information published by the German National Library:

The German National Library lists this publication in the National Bibliography; detailed bibliographic data are available on the Internet at http://dnb.dnb.de.

ISBN: 9783346801661
This book is also available as an ebook.

© GRIN Publishing GmbH
Nymphenburger Straße 86
80636 München

Print and binding: Books on Demand GmbH, Norderstedt, Germany
Printed on acid-free paper from responsible sources.

The present work has been carefully prepared. Nevertheless, authors and publishers do not incur liability for the correctness of information, notes, links and advice as well as any printing errors.

GRIN web shop: https://www.grin.com/document/1320365

Table of Contents

CHAPTER ONE: Introduction

1.1 Background of the Study

The leaves, flowers, stems, roots and other components derived from plants have

been reported to be effective antibacterial agents. Traditional herbalists in Nigeria

use herbal preparations to treat various types of ailments, including diarrhea,

urinary tract infections (UTIs), typhoid fever and skin diseases (Sofowora, 2010).

The World Health Organization (WHO, 2010) survey indicated that about 70- 80%

of the world's population particularly in developed countries rely on non-

conventional medicines mainly of herbal origins for their primary health care. This

is because herbal medicines are accessible and cheap (Sofowora, 2010). With the

increased usage of herbal preparations in Nigeria, the safety, efficacy and quality

of these medicines have been an important concern for health authorities and

health professionals (Adeleye *et al.*, 2015).

Antibiotic resistant bacteria have been a source of an ever increasing therapeutic

problem (Sheikh *et al.*, 2013). Drug resistant infectious microorganisms have

become an important public health concern. Aside from the public health threat

drug resistant microorganisms pose, research into newer antibiotics to overcome

resistant microbes is usually very expensive and contributes to the higher costs of

health care (Adeleye *et al.*, 2015).

Resistant bacteria strains may develop almost anywhere particularly in a pressurized environment containing previously non-resistant bacteria strains as contaminants. One of such environments can be herbal medicinal products (HMPs). Herbal medicinal products have been previously implicated as a pool for such contaminations (Esimone *et al.*, 2017). It is of utmost importance to monitor and ascertain the microbial purity of HMPs given the huge medical and economic implications of any such microbial contamination especially with multiple drug resistant strains. Such surveillance will help to identify microbial contamination of herbal products and slow down or prevent the emergence of drug-resistant strains (Odimegwu *et al.*, 2011).

1.2 Aim of the Study

The aim of this study is to determine the efficacy of herbal mixtures on some selected bacteria, *Staphylococcus aureus* and *Streptococcus pyogene*

1.3 Objectives of the Study

The objectives of this study include:

- To determine the antibacterial efficacy of herbal mixtures on some selected bacteria, *Staphylococcus aureus* and *Streptococcus pyogene*
- To determine the minimum inhibitory concentration of herbal mixtures some selected bacteria, against *Staphylococcus aureus* and *Streptococcus pyogene*.

3

- To determine the minimum bactericidal concentration of herbal mixtures some selected bacteria, against *Staphylococcus aureus* and *Streptococcus pyogene*

CHAPTER TWO: Literature review

2.1 Medicinal Plants in Nigeria with Antimicrobial Activities

Despite the success of antibiotic discovery, infectious diseases are consistently ranked second among causes of death worldwide (Pavithra *et al.*, 2010). The pursuit of new compounds that have therapeutic potential for infectious diseases with no existing remedy such as Lassa fever and others focuses mainly on plants as the best reservoir of drug compounds. The microbial resistance to antibiotics is among the significant problems in the twenty-first century and has necessitated the need for a continuous search for more potent and safe therapeutic agents (Chikezie *et al.*, 2015).

2.1.1 Antibacterial Activity

Tuberculosis (TB) is a life-threatening disease caused by various Mycobacterium species and has been ranked among the leading causes of human death in the developing nations (Okwuosa *et al.*, 2012). In 2013, WHO reported that approximately 8.6 million people incurred TB and 1.3 million died from it, with an estimated 450,000 new cases of multidrug-resistant TB worldwide. Chronic cough is a feature of many common respiratory diseases with the percentage of global occurrence in Oceania (18.1%), Europe (12.7%), America (11.0%), Asia (4.4%), and Africa (2.3%) (Aiyeloja and Bello, 2016). Diarrhea is a killer disease;

according to 2015 observatory data of WHO, the occurrence of childhood mortality in developing nations due to diarrhoeal disease between 9% and 34%. Many enteric bacterial pathogens are responsible for diarrhea, which include bacteria such as *Vibrio cholera*, *Campylobacter jejuni*, *Helicobacter pylori*, *Salmonella typhi* or paratyphi, *Shigella flexneri*, *Clostridium difficile*, and Shiga toxin-producing *Escherichia coli*. Findings of Ogbonnia *et al.* (2018) and Oladele *et al.* (2019) stated that the root and leaf extracts of *Terminalia glaucescens* show appreciable activity against *E. coli* and *S. typhi*. The methanol extracts of three Nigerian medicinal plants have antimicrobial activity against five clinical bacterial isolates comprising two Gram-positive bacteria (*Bacillus subtilis* and *Staphylococcus aureus*) and three Gram-negative bacteria (*Pseudomonas aeruginosa*, *E. coli*, and Klebsiella pneumonia) organisms (Chikezie *et al.*, 2015). Acetone and ethanol extracts of bark of *Azadirachta indica* (A. Juss.), at a concentration of 25–400 mg/ml, showed significant antibacterial activity on all 14 strains of multidrug-resistant *Salmonella typhi* with zone diameter of 18–31 mm (Okpe *et al.*, 2016). An investigation of the activity of aqueous and ethanolic extracts of *Zingiber officinale* and *Allium sativum* extracts on selected foodborne pathogens (*Salmonella* species, *Bacillus cereus*, *E. coli,* and *S. aureus*) showed multidrug resistance. *E. coli* sensitive to aqueous extracts, but *S. aureus* and *Salmonella* species were sensitive to ethanol extracts (Ola-Fadunsin and Ademola,

6

2014). The alcoholic extracts from the leaves of two *Diospyros* spp. (*D. barteri*

and *D. monbuttensis*) showed potent antibacterial activity against a wide range of

Gram-positive and Gram-negative bacteria, while two fungal species investigated

in the study, *Aspergillus niger* and *Candida albicans*, were resistant to the extracts

of both *Diospyros* spp. (Suleiman *et al.*, 2018). The result of in vitro study of

water, methanol, chloroform, and petroleum ether extracts of Senna alata flowers,

which examined antimicrobial properties at a final concentration of 500 µg/mL,

showed antimicrobial activities against clinical isolates of *S. aureus*, *C. albicans*,

E. coli, *Proteus vulgaris*, *P. aeruginosa*, and *B. subtilis* (Omotoyinbo and Sani,

2015). *Heeria insignis* O. Ktze, a member of the family *Anacardiaceae*, is an

indigenous African shrub used in the treatment of diarrhea, *schistosomiasis*, and

venereal diseases. The methanol and dichloromethane extracts of the leaves of *H.*

insignis possessed antibacterial and antidiarrheal activities, while methanol showed

a more significant antibacterial activity than dichloromethane (Keyal *et al.*, 2016).

However, aqueous extracts of the stem bark of *Spondias mombin* have outstanding

anthelmintic activity at low concentrations (Uzodinma, 2013). Preliminary

investigation of the in vitro vibriocidal activities of three medicinal plants

(traditional Ogi-tutu, *Psidium guajava*, and *Vernonia amygdalina*), using agar cup

diffusion assay, showed that *V. amygdalina* has the highest ameliorative effects in

the deterrence and cure of *V. cholerae* infection (Suleyman and Alangaden, 2016).

Moreover, a study has revealed the antibacterial property of *T. vulgaris* on multiple antibiotic-resistant *Vibrio fluvialis* and *Vibrio parahaemolyticus* isolated from shrimps using agar diffusion method (Suleyman and Alangaden, 2016). The examination of *Argemone mexicana* L. for antimicrobial activity showed that the aerial and root extracts inhibited *B. subtilis* and K. pneumoniae, but *P. aeruginosa* and *S. aureus* were not prone to the aerial and root extracts.

In Nigerian ethnomedicine, Annona senegalensis Pers. (Annonaceae) has been used for the treatment of infectious diseases. Okokon *et al.* (2017) investigated A. senegalensis using the GC-MS and agar-well-diffusion method and found that lipophilic fraction and kaurenoic acid from A. senegalensis root bark showed potent antibacterial activity. Furthermore, the results of in vivo and in vitro model investigations of the antidiarrheal properties of the stem bark extract of A. senegalensis using mice and isolated rabbit jejunum showed maximum inhibition at a dose of 10 mg/kg. At the same time, intestinal transit time decreased at concentrations of 0.2–3.2 mg/ml, and the extract lessened spontaneous contractions of the jejunum (Cheesman *et al.*, 2017). Ficus exasperata Vahl-Holl (Moraceae) leaves in West Africa are used for the treatment of infectious diseases and inflammatory conditions. However, a more thorough phytochemical analysis of the ethnomedicinal uses of F. exasperata has identified new compounds: apigenin C-8 glucoside, isoquercitrin-6- O-4-hydroxybenzoate, and quercetin-3-O-β-rhamnoside, as some of the constituents of this plant that inhibited the growth of Gram-positive organisms only (Hassan *et al.*, 2016).

2.2 Antimalarial Activity

Malaria, a significant threat to global health, is responsible for the death of millions of people predominantly in sub-Saharan Africa. The occurrence of multidrug-resistant malaria parasites has triggered efforts to develop combined formulations (such as artemether-lumefantrine and sulfadoxine-pyrimethamine) and continuous research toward discovering better therapeutics. An in vitro study by Oladele (2018) on the sensitivity pattern of *Plasmodium falciparum* to *Diospyros monbuttensis* ("Egun eja"), *Momordica charantia* ("Ejirin"), and *Morinda lucida* ("Oruwo") recorded the lowest antiplasmodial activity with the ethanolic extract of *M. lucida* while *D. monbuttensis* recorded the highest activity. Oladele (2018), investigated the antiplasmodial activity of crude n-hexane and ethanolic extracts of *M. oleifera* seeds using the cold extraction method and found the highest parasite inhibition activity in crude ethanolic extract. Besides, *Landolphia owariensis P. Beauv.*, a member of the family *Apocynaceae*, is used in southeast Nigeria for the treatment of malaria. A study has shown that methanol fractions of *L. owariensis* leaf in early, established, and residual infections in

9

Plasmodium berghei-infected albino mice have the most significant antiplasmodial activity in all the models carried out, due to alkaloids, flavonoids, saponins, and tannins present in the fractions (Butler and Buss, 2016). *Allamanda cathartica* and *Bixa orellana* are antimalarial plants (Handa *et al.*, 2018). Moreover, *Alchornea laxiflora* (Benth.), a member of the family *Euphorbiaceae*, is used traditionally in the treatment of malaria in Nigeria. Furthermore, the study has shown that root extract *A. laxiflora* exerted significant antimalarial activity against *P. berghei* infection while ethyl acetate fraction exerted the highest activity against chloroquine-sensitive (Pf3D7) and -resistant (PfINDO) strains of *P. falciparum* infection in mice (Conrad *et al.*, 2013). *Enantia chlorantha* has significant utilization in traditional medicine for the treatment of several diseases which include malaria. However, another study has suggested that oral administration of *E. chlorantha* at relatively high doses may produce severe toxic effects (Ozioma and Chinwe, 2019). A study on the acute and subacute toxicity of the medicinal plant *E. chlorantha* carried out in mice showed a mean lethal dose (LD50) of 0.7 g·kg−1 for ethanolic but 43.65 g·kg−1 for aqueous preparations (Ivana *et al.*, 2016). *Cajanus cajan* (L.) is a member of the family Fabaceae and possesses antimalarial properties. The result of the in vitro investigation of crude methanolic extract of C. cajan leaves, using the multiresistant strain of *P. falciparum* (K1) and combination of chromatographic techniques, identified cajachalcone (2′,6′-

10

dihydroxy-4-methoxy chalcone) from the ethyl acetate fraction, as one of the biologically active constituents (Subramaniyan et al., 2016).

2.3   Antifungal Activity

Infections caused by fungi are termed fungal infections or mycoses. Fungal infections have been considered a serious health problem and life-threatening diseases in recent years, especially in immunodeficiency conditions (Ogbole et al., 2018) Severe fungal diseases result from other health challenges such as human immunodeficiency virus (HIV), asthma, cancer, organ transplantation, and corticosteroid treatments (Okigbo et al., 2019). In Nigeria, fungal infections (cryptococcal antigenemia, subclinical histoplasmosis) have been implicated in HIV/AIDS patients and neonatal intensive care babies (Ajaiyeoba et al., 2013). In Cameroun, esophageal candidiasis, cryptococcal meningitis, Pneumocystis pneumonia, disseminated histoplasmosis, and invasive aspergillosis were prevalent in adults, while tinea capitis prevalent among school children (Odelola and Okorosobo, 2010). In Mozambique, disseminated Emergomyces and recurrent Candida vulvovaginitis were common among HIV patients (Jebashree et al., 2011). Some hospitalized patients are at risk of contracting fungal infections (Vambe et al., 2018). Besides, emerging and reemerging fungal infections due to recent therapies for autoimmune and cancer-related diseases (hematopoietic stem cell

11

transplant) are becoming public health concern (Lockhart and Guarner, 2019). Different parts of *Calotropis procera*, a flowering plant that belongs to the family *Asclepiadaceous*, have been utilized in traditional medicine for the treatment of infections which include eczema, cutaneous infections, leprosy, and syphilis, as well as malaria. In a study on antifungal activity of *C. procera*, there complete inhibition of *Microsporum* and *Trichophyton* species after ten days of inoculation with water extract at different concentrations (Ugboko *et al.*, 2016). Crude methanolic extract of *Spondias mombin* (bark and leaves) found to exhibit anti-candidal effects with diameters of 11.00 ± 0.47 mm and 15.00 ± 0.47 mm, respectively. The extracts have varying degrees of phytochemical compositions such as terpenoids, alkaloids, glycosides, saponin, and flavonoids (Agbaje and Onabanjo, 2010). *Psidium guajava* extracts were active on *Candida albicans* isolates from caries infected patients (Adeniyi *et al.*, 2015). Additionally, *Alchornea laxiflora* leaf extracts have antibacterial and antifungal activities due to flavonoids, alkaloids, saponins, tannins, and reducing sugars as major phytochemicals (Aiyegoro and Okoh, 2019).

2.4 Antiviral Activity

Human immunodeficiency virus type 1 (HIV-1) encodes reverse transcriptase which functions in the process of the viral genome reverse transcription, a

12

fundamental step in the HIV-1 replication cycle and promising target in the antiretroviral drug development (Tiwari *et al.*, 2011). A study conducted in Nigeria by Taiwo and Igbeneghu (2014) on the antiviral activities of 27 medicinal plant extracts, belonging to 26 different plant species, against echovirus 7, 13, and 19 serotypes (E7, E13, and E19, respectively) revealed the highest antiviral activity from methanolic extract of *Macaranga barteri* leaves on E7 and E9, respectively, followed by *Ageratum conyzoides* leaves extract on E7 and E19 and *Mondia whitei* leaves extract on E7 and E19. In China, *Rheum palmatum* and *Rheum officinale* extracts along with their main single isolated constituents' anthraquinone derivatives inhibited both HIV-1 reverse transcriptase-associated DNA polymerase (RDDP) and ribonuclease H activities (Nayak *et al.*, 2011). The screening of some plants showed antiretroviral activities. For instance, *Ancistrocladus korupensis* and *Ancistrocladus congolensis* produced michellamine A and B, *Ancistrocladus congolensis* (Boyd *et al.*, 2016).

CHAPTER THREE: Material and Method

3.1   Study Area

This study was carried out at the Microbiology laboratory, University of Abuja, Gwagwalada FCT-Abuja- Nigeria. Gwagwalada is one of the five municipal Councils of the Federal Capital Territory of Nigeria, together with Abaji, Kuje, Bwari, and Kwali; the FCT also includes the City of Abuja. Gwagwalada is also the name of the main town in the Local Government Area, which has an area of 1,043 km² and a population of 157,770 at the 2016 census (Awowole and Francis, 2017). Gwagwalada is where the University of Abuja is located.

3.2   Preparation and Sterilization media

Media used include Nutrient agar and Mueller Hinton agar. All media was prepared according to the manufacturers' instructions. Nutrient Agar used for this study was prepared according to the manufacturer specification. Seven (7) g of Nutrient agar was weighed and suspended in 250 ml of distilled water. It was shaken carefully so as to dissolve completely; cotton wool was wrapped in aluminum foil and was used to cover the mouth of the conical flask which was transfer to the autoclave for sterilization. It was autoclaved for 15 minutes at 121 °C. After autoclaving the conical flask was placed on the work bench and allowed to cool to 47 °C before dispensing about 20ml was poured into sterile petri dishes and allowed to solidify.

3.3   Collection and Identifications of Bacterial Isolates

Samples of clinical isolates of *Staphylococcus aureus* and *Streptococcus pyogene* was collected from the University of Abuja Teaching Hospital Gwagwalada and brought to Microbiology laboratory, University of Abuja FCT-Abuja for further identifications. The isolate was characterized and identified on the basis of the cultural, morphological and biochemical characteristics.

3.3.1 Cultural Characteristics

The bacterial colonies was observed for size, texture, colour, shape, colony surface and edges/margin.

3.3.2 Biochemical Tests

The biochemical characteristics used are; catalase test, oxidase test, urease test, coagulase test.

3.3.2.1 Coagulase Test

A drop of distilled water was placed on a clean grease free slide and a colony of the test organism was picked and emulsified on the drop of water to make a thick

15

suspension. A loopful of plasma was added to the suspension and mixed gently to observe for clumping of the organism within 10 seconds (Cheesbrough, 2006).

3.3.2.2   Catalase Test

Three (3) ml of hydrogen peroxide solution was dispensed in a sterile test tube and several colonies of 18 h culture of the test organism was picked and immersed in the hydrogen peroxide solution using a glass rod. It was observed for immediate bubbling which indicated positive result (Cheesbrouhg, 2006).

3.3.2.3   Methyl Red Test

This test was carried out according to Cheesbrough (2006). The test organism was inoculated in sterile peptone water and incubated for 24 hours to obtain a broth culture. Prepared 5% peptone water plus 0.5 g of D glucose plus 0.5g of potassium pallidium was sterilized and allowed to cool and 2.5 ml of the broth culture was added and incubated at 4°C for 24 hours. On addition of methyl red, the appearance of red color indicates positive reaction for methyl red.

3.4   Collection of Herbal Products

A liquid herbal mixture of a known manufacturer's marketed in Gwagwalada FCT Abuja were randomly selected and purchased for the efficacy against selected bacteria, *Staphylococcus aureus* and *Streptococcus pyogene*. The herbal mixture was coded as KC and stored at 4°C until used.

The composition of the herbal mixture is represented below:

Aloe vulgaris (Aloe vera),

Capensis hydrostis,

Canadensis enchinacea,

Angostifolia, and Honey.

3.4.1 Preparation of Herbal Products

The purchased liquid herbal products were concentrated on the water bath for seven (7) days to obtain various extracts and properly labeled until needed for use.

3.5 Determination of Antimicrobial Activity

Antibacterial activity of the liquid herbal mixture was evaluated by the agar well diffusion method as described by Charteris *et al.* (2010). The bacteria (*Staphylococcus aureus* and *Streptococcus pyogene*) culture was adjusted to 0.5Mc.farland standard and poured onto freshly prepared Mueller Hinton agar plates. A sterile cork borer was used to make a well (6 mm in diameter) on the MHA plates. Aliquots of 100 μL (i.e 0.1ml) of the extracts dilutions, reconstituted in distilled water at concentrations of 100, 200, 400 and 500 mg/ml, was applied in each of the wells in the culture plates previously seeded with the test organisms. The cultures was incubated at 37°C for 24 hours. A well was made in each of the culture plates and filled with 20 μl of 10 mg/ml of amoxicillin as control.

Antimicrobial activity was determined by measuring the zone of inhibition around each well (excluding the diameter of the well). All the experiments were carrying out in triplicate.

3.5.1 Determination of Minimum Inhibitory Concentration (MIC)

The Minimum Inhibitory Concentration (MIC) of the extracts was determined for each of the plant extract against the test organism (*Staphylococcus aureus* and *Streptococcus pyogene*) in test tubes. To 0.5 ml of varying concentrations of the extracts (100, 200, 400 and 500 mg/ml) in test tubes, Nutrient broth (2ml) was added and then a loopful of the test organism, previously diluted to 0.5 Mc Farland turbidity standard, was introduced. The procedure was repeated on the test organisms using the standard antibiotic (ciprofloxacin). A tube containing Nutrient broth only was seeded with the test organisms, as described above, to serve as control. The culture tubes were then incubated at 37^0C for 24 h. After incubation the tubes was then examined for microbial growth by observing for turbidity (Bauer *et al.*, 2016). All the experiments were carried out in triplicates.

3.5.2 Determination of Minimum Bactericidal Concentration (MBC)

To determine the MBC, for each set of test tubes in the MIC determination, a loopful of broth was collected from those tubes that did not show any bacterial growth in the MIC and inoculated on sterile Nutrient agar by streaking. All the plates was then incubated at 37°C for 24h. After incubation period, the concentration at which no visible growth occurred on the plate was noted as the Minimum Bactericidal Concentration (MBC) (Cheesebrough, 2016). All the experiments was carried out in triplicates.

3.6 Statistical Analysis

The statistical analysis was determined using one way Analysis of Variance (ANOVA) from Ms Excel Statistics. Test applied was F-test statistic at p= 0.05.

CHAPTER FOUR: Results

4.1 Antibacterial Effect of Herbal Mixtures

Table 1 below shows the result of zone of inhibitions of Aqueous extracts of the herbal mixtures as described in the material and methods is presented. The zone diameter of inhibition in millimeter of Aqueous extracts of herbal mixture at concentration of 500 mg/ml against *Staphylococcus aureus* shows that Herbal mixture met the standard of the antibiotic used as the positive control (Chloramphenicol) with 25.0±1.0 mm each. Meanwhile *Streptococcus pyogene* had significant zone diameter of inhibition (24mm against the herbal mixtures) at concentration of 500mg/ml.

Table 1: Zone Diameter of Inhibition (ZDI) in millimeter of Aqueous

Test Isolates	Concentration in mg/ml			
	100	200	400	500
Streptococcus pyogene	18.0±1.5	17.0±1.0	21.0±1.0	24.0±1.0
Staphylococus aureus	20.0±1.0	19.0±0.5	23.0±0.5	25.0±1.0
Chloramphenicol	20.0±1.5	22.0±1.5	23.0±1.0	25.0±1.0

Each value represents mean ± standard deviation of duplicate values.

4.2 Minimum Inhibitory Concentrations of the Herbal Mixture Extracts

The extracts of the herbal mixture had the minimum inhibition concentration (MIC) of 200 mg/ml against *Staphylococcus aureus* and which correlate with the control (Chloramphenicol), while the MIC of 400 mg/ml against *Streptococcus pyogene* respectively as seen in Table 2.

Table 2: Minimum Inhibitory Concentration of the Aqueous Extracts against *Streptococcus pyogene* and *Staphylococcus aureus*

Test Isolates	Concentration in mg/ml			
	100	200	400	500
Streptococcus pyogene	+	+	MIC	-
Staphylococus aureus	+	MIC	-	-
Chloramphenicol	MIC	-	-	-

Key: + =Present, - =Absent

4.4   Minimum Bactericidal Concentrations of the Plant Extracts

The Minimum bactericidal concentration of the extracts shows that the herbal mixture have the least value of 400 mg/ml which correlates with the standard antibiotic (Chloramphenicol) used as control against *Streptococcus pyogene*. Similarly from the same Table 2, the Herbal mixture had MBC of 400 mg/ml which also correlates with the standard antibiotics drug (Chloramphenicol) as seen in Table 3.

Table 3: Minimum Bactericidal Concentration of the Aqueous Extracts against *Streptococcus pyogene* and *Staphylococcus aureus*

Test Isolates	100	Concentration in mg/ml		
		200	400	500
Streptococcus pyogene	+	+	MBC	-
Staphylococus aureus	+	+	MBC	-
Chloramphenicol	+	+	MBC	-

Key: + =Present, - =Absent

CHAPTER FIVE: Discussions and Conclusions

5.1 Discussions

This study revealed that the antibacterial activity of the herbal mixtures against all the test organisms increased as the concentration increased. The mixture had antibacterial effects on all the test organisms but the effect of the control (Chloramphenicol) was significantly higher ($P< 0.05$). This is also in agreement with Achi (2016) who reported similar activity. In this study, the common conventional antibiotic Chloramphenicol employed exhibited comparative higher zones of inhibition as compared to all the extracts except.

The zone diameter of inhibition in millimeter of Aqueous extracts of Herbal mixture at concentration of 500 mg/ml against *Staphylococcus aureus* shows that Herbal mixture met the standard of the antibiotic used as the positive control (Chloramphenicol) with 25.0 ± 1.0 mm each. Meanwhile *Streptococcus pyogene* had significant zone diameter of inhibition (24 mm) at concentration of 500mg/ml.

This agrees with Agatemor (2019) which reported the Antimicrobial activity of aqueous and ethanol extracts of nine Nigerian spices against four food borne bacteria. The zones of inhibitions of the herbal mixture extracts against *Streptococcus pyogene* at 200 mg/ml were appreciable. The zone diameter of inhibition in millimeter of Aqueous extracts of Herbal mixture at concentration of 500 mg/ml against *Streptococcus pyogene* shows that Herbal mixture almost met the standard of the antibiotic used as the positive control (Chloramphenicol) with 25.0±1.0 mm each. This agrees with Akinyemi et al. (2014) on the Screening of some medicinal plants for anti Salmonella activity. Minimum inhibitory concentration is a quantitative assay and provides more information on the potency of the compounds present in the extracts. Thus, the minimum inhibitory concentration values of crude extracts of the six medicinal herbs were determined so as to demonstrate the potency of the extracts against test organisms.

The herbal mixture had the minimum inhibition concentration (MIC) of 200mg/ml against Staphylococcus aureus and which correlate with the control (Chloramphenicol), while MIC of 400 mg/ml against Streptococcus pyogene. This agrees with the findings of Sofowora, (2013). This also agrees with the findings of Nweze et al., (2014). The least minimum inhibitory concentration of the herbal mixture extract against the isolate in question. The Minimum bactericidal concentration of the extracts shows that the least value of 400 mg/ml which correlates with the standard antibiotic (Chloramphenicol) used as control against Streptococcus pyogene while it had 500 mg/ml as MBC against Salmonella tyhi as seen in Table 2. Similarly from the same Table 2, the herbal mixture had MBC of 250 mg/ml which also correlates with the standard antibiotics drug (Chloramphenicol). This also agrees with the findings of Akinyemi et al. (2014). It has further confirmed that the extracts could be use for the treatment of various infections caused by the pathogens. The results lend credence to the folkloric use of this plant in treating microbial infections and shows that Herbal mixture extracts could be exploited for new potent antibiotics.

5.2 Conclusion

The aqueous herbal mixture extract in this study has high activity against bacteria strains as. Traditionally medicine plants decoction are taken in combination and at high dose, this may explain the low and moderate activity observed. In this study, the minimum inhibitory concentration of all the plant extracts shown that there was no activity against *Staphylococcus aureus* and *Streptococcus pyogene* at low concentration of 100 mg/ml thus treating ailments caused by pathogenic strains of test organisms at such concentration will not work. The results validate the ethnobotanical use of the studied medicinal plants used among the coastal people of Nigeria.

5.3 Recommendation

Since the extracts are potent against bacterial isolates as seen in this study then it is worth recommending the extracts be tested against a wide range of bacteria.

- Analysis and isolation of the compounds present as well as determination of their bioactivity of the pure compounds should also be done. Such an effort could lead to identification of a new range of compounds for management of bacterial infections.

- Bioassay of combinations of plant extracts that exhibited moderate and low activity should be carried out to establish any synergism between them.

REFERENCES

Adebiyi, O. E. and Abatan, M. O. (2013). "Phytochemical and acute toxicity of ethanolic extract of *Enantia chlorantha* (olive) stem bark in albino rats". *Interdisciplinary Toxicology*, 6(3):145–151.

Adeleye, I.A., Okogi, G. and Ojo, E.O. (2015). Microbial contamination of herbal preparations in Lagos, Nigeria. *Journal of Health and Nutrition*, 23(3): 296-297.

Adeniyi, B. A., Ayepola, O.O. and Adu, F. D. (2015). "The antiviral activity of leaves of *Eucalyptus camaldulensis* (dehn) and *Eucalyptus torelliana* (R. muell)," *Pakistan Journal of Pharmaceutical Sciences*, 28(5): 1773–1776.

Agbaje, E. O. and Onabanjo, A. O. (2010). "Toxicological study of the extracts of anti-malarial medicinal plant *Enantia chlorantha*". *Central African Journal of Medicine*, 40(3): 71–73.

Agunloye, O. M. and Oboh, G. (2018). "Effect of different processing methods on antihypertensive property and antioxidant activity of sandpaper leaf (*Ficus exasperata*) extracts". *Journal of Dietary Supplements*, 15(6): 871–883.

Agunu, A., Ahmadu, A. A., Afolabi, S. O., Yaro, A. U., Ehinmidu, J. O. and Mohammed, Z. (2011). "Evaluation of the antibacterial and antidiarrhoeal activities of *Heeria insignis*". *Indian Journal of Pharmaceutical Sciences*, 73(3): 328–332.

Aiyegoro, O. A. and Okoh, A. I. (2019). "Use of bioactive plant products in combination with standard antibiotics: implications in antimicrobial chemotherapy". *Journal of Medicinal Plants Research*, 3(13):1147–1152.

Aiyeloja, A. A. and. Bello, O. A. (2016). "Ethnobotanical potentials of common herbs in Nigeria: a case study of Enugu state". *Educational Research and Reviews*, 1: 16–22.

Ajaiyeoba, E.O., Ogbole, O. O., Abiodun, O. O., Ashidi, J. S., Houghton, P. J. and Wright, C. W. (2013). "Cajachalcone: an antimalarial compound from *Cajanus cajan* leaf extract". *Journal of Parasitology Research*, 20(13):5.

Ajayi, O., Awala, S., Ogunleye, A., Okogbue, F. and Olaleye, B. F. (2016). "Antimicrobial screening and phytochemical analysis of *Elaeis guineensis* (ewe igi ope) against salmonella strains". *British Journal of Pharmaceutical Research*, 10(3): 1–9.

Akinpelu, D. A., Abioye, E. O., Aiyegoro, O. A., Akinpelu, O. F.V.V. and Okoh, A. I. (2015). "Evaluation of antibacterial and antifungal properties of *Alchornea laxiflora* (benth.) pax. and hoffman". *Evidence-Based Complementary and Alternative Medicine*, 2015:13.

Baba, H. and Onanuga, A. (2011). "Preliminary phytochemical screening and antimicrobial evaluation of three medicinal plants used in Nigeria". *African Journal of Traditional, Complementary and Alternative Medicines*, 8(4): 20-11.

Boyd, G., Steinert, C., Feineis, D., Mudogo, V., Betzin, J. and Scheller, C. (2016). "HIV-inhibitory michellamine-type dimeric naphthylisoquinoline alkaloids from the central african liana *Ancistrocladus congolensis*". *Phytochemistry*, 128:71–81.

Butler, M. S. and Buss, A. D. (2016). "Natural products—the future scaffolds for novel antibiotics?". *Biochemical Pharmacology*, 71(7): 919–929.

Cheesman, M. J., Ilanko, A., Blonk, B. and Cock, I. E. (2017). "Developing new antimicrobial therapics: are synergistic combinations of plant extracts/compounds with conventional antibiotics the solution?". *Pharmacognosy Reviews*, 11(22): 57.

Chikezie, P. C., Ibegbulem, C. O. and Mbagwu, F. N. (2015). "Bioactive principles from medicinal plants". *Research Journal of Phytochemistry*, 9(3): 88–115.

Conrad, O. A., Dike, I. P. and Agbara, U. (2013). "In vivo antioxidant assessment of two antimalarial plants-*Allamamda cathartica* and *Bixa orellana*". *Asian Pacific Journal of Tropical Biomedicine*, 3(5): 388–394.

Corona, A., Masaoka, T., Tocco, G., Tramontano, E. and Le Grice, S. F. (2013). "Active site and allosteric inhibitors of the ribonuclease H activity of HIV reverse transcriptase". *Future Medicinal Chemistry*, 5(18): 2127–2139.

Esimone, C.O., Oleghe, P.O., Ibezim, E.C. and Iroha, I.R. (2017). Susceptibility-resistance profile of micro-organisms isolated from herbal medicine products sold in Nigeria. *African Journal Biotechnology,* 6(24): 2766–2775.

Esposito, F., Carli, I. and Del Vecchio, C. (2016). "Sennoside A, derived from the traditional Chinese medicine plant rheum L., is a new dual HIV-1 inhibitor effective on HIV-1 replication". *Phytomedicine*, 23(12): 1383–1391.

Ezike, A. C., Okonkwo, C. H., Akah, P. A., Okoye, T.C. and Nworu, C.S. (2016). "*Landolphia owariensis* leaf extracts reduce parasitemia in *Plasmodium berghei*-infected mice". *Pharmaceutical Biology*, 54(10): 2017–2025.

Gbolade, A. A. and Adeyemi, A. A. (2018). "Anthelmintic activities of three medicinal plants from Nigeria". *Fitoterapia*, 79(3):223–225.

Handa, S. S., Khanuja, S. P. S., Longo, G. and Rakesh, D. D. (2018). *Extraction Technologies for Medicinal and Aromatic Plants.* International Centre for Science and High Technology, Trieste, Italy, pp. 2-8.

Hassan, S. T. S., Berchov´a, K., Majerov´a, M., Pokorn´a, M. and ˇSvajdlenka, E.(2016). "In vitro synergistic effect of *Hibiscus sabdariffa* aqueous extract in combination with standard antibiotics against *Helicobacter pylori* clinical isolates". *Pharmaceutical Biology*, 54(9): 1736–1740.

Hemaiswarya, S., Kruthiventi, A. K. and Doble, M. (2018). "Synergism between natural products and antibiotics against infectious diseases". *Phytomedicine*, 15(8): 639–652.

Ivana, B. S., Mateus, L. B. P., Antonio, D. V. and Riad, N. Y. (2016). "Antibacterial activity of Brazilian amazon plant extracts". *Brazilian Journal of Infectious Diseases*, 10(6): 2-6.

Jebashree, H. S., Kingsley, S. J., Sathish, E. S. and Devapriya, D. (2011). "Antimicrobial activity of few medicinal plants against clinically isolated human cariogenic pathogens—an in vitro study". *ISRN Dentistry*, 20(11): 6.

Kennedy, D. O. and Wightman, E. L. (2011). "Herbal extracts and phytochemicals: plant secondary metabolites and the enhancement of human brain function". *Advances in Nutrition*, 2(1): 32–50.

Keyal, U., Huang, X. and Bhatta, A. K. (2016). "Antifungal effect of plant extract and essential oil," *Chinese Journal of Integrative Medicine*, 23.

Khan, R., Islam, B. and Akram, B. (2019). "Antimicrobial activity of five herbal extracts against multi drug resistant (MDR) strains of bacteria and fungus of clinical origin," *Molecules*, 14(2): 586–597.

Lockhart, S. R. and Guarner, J. (2019). "Emerging and reemerging fungal infections," in *Seminars in Diagnostic Pathology*, WB Saunders, Philadelphia, PA, USA, pp. 177–181.

Maitera, O. N., Louis, H., Oyebanji, O.O. and Anumah, A. O. (2018). "Investigation of tannin content in *Diospyros mespiliformis* extract using various extraction solvents". *Journal of Analytical and Pharmaceutical Research*, 7(1): 2-18.

Meskin, M. S. (2012). *Phytochemicals in Nutrition and Health*, CRC Press, Boca Raton, FL, USA.

Nayak, B., Liu, R. H., Berrios, J. D. J., Tang, J. and Derito, C. (2011). "Bioactivity of antioxidants in extruded products prepared from purple potato and dry pea flours". *Journal of Agricultural and Food Chemistry*, 59(15): 8233–8243.

Nayak, B., Liu, R. H. and Tang, J. (2015). "Effect of processing on phenolic antioxidants of fruits, vegetables, and grains-a review". *Critical Reviews in Food Science and Nutrition*, 55(7): 887–918.

Odelola, H. A. and Okorosobo, V. I. (2010). "Preliminary investigation of in-vitro antimicrobial activity of two Nigerian diospyros species (ebenaceae)". *African Journal of Medicine and Medical Sciences*, 17(3):167–170.

Odimegwu, D.C., Oleghe, P.O., Udofia, E. and Esimone, C.O. (2011). Multi-drug-resistant bacteria isolates recovered from herbal medicinal preparations in a southern Nigerian setting. *Journal of Rural Tropical Public Health*, 10: 70 - 75.

Ogbole, O. O., Akinleye, T. E., Segun, P. A., Faleye, T. C. and Adeniji, A. J. (2018). "In vitro antiviral activity of twenty-seven medicinal plant extracts from southwest Nigeria against three serotypes of echoviruses". *Virology Journal*, 15(1): 110.

Ogbonnia, S., Adekunle, A. A., Bosa, M. K. and Enwuru, V.N. (2018). "Evaluation of acute and subacute toxicity of *Alstonia congensis* engler (apocynaceae) bark and *Xylopia aethiopica* (dunal) *A. rich* (Annonaceae) fruits mixtures used in the treatment of diabetes". *African Journal of Biotechnology*, 247: 188–192.

Okigbo, R. N., Anuagasi, C. L. and Amadi, J. E. (2019). "Advances in selected medicinal and aromatic plants indigenous to Africa". *Journal of Medicinal Plants Research*, 3(2): 86–95.

Okokon, J. E., Augustine, N. B. and Mohanakrishnan, D. (2017). "Antimalarial, antiplasmodial and analgesic activities of root extract of *Alchornea laxiflora*". *Pharmaceutical Biology*, 55(1): 1022–1031.

Okoye, T. C., Akah, P. A., Okoli, C. O., Ezike, A. C., Omeje, E. O. and Odoh, U. E. (2012). "Antimicrobial effects of a lipophilic fraction and kaurenoic acid isolated from the root bark extracts of *Annona senegalensis*". *Evidence-Based Complementary and Alternative Medicine*, 20(12): 10.

Okpe, O., Habila, N., Ikwebe, J., Upev, V.A., Okoduwa, S. I. R. and Isaac, O. T. (2016). "Antimalarial potential of *Carica papaya* and *Vernonia amygdalina* in mice infected with *Plasmodium berghei*". *Journal of Tropical Medicine*, 20(16): 6.

Okwuosa, O. M., Chukwura, E. I. and Chukwuma, G. O. (2012). "Phytochemical and antifungal activities of Uvaria. Chamae leaves and roots, *Spondias mombin* leaves and bark and *Combretum racemosum* leaves". *African Journal of Medicine and Medical Sciences*, 41:99–103.

Oladele, R. O. (2018). *Current Status of Serious Fungal Infections in Nigeria*, the University of Manchester, Manchester, UK, pp.2-18.

Oladele, R. O., Osaigbovo, I.I., Ayanlowo, O.O., Otu, A.A. and Hoenigl, M. (2019). "The role of medical mycology societies in combating invasive fungal infections in low- and middleincome countries: a Nigerian model". *Mycoses*, 62(1): 16–21.

Oladosu, I. A., Balogun, S. O. and L. Zhi-Qiang, L. (2015). "Chemical constituents of *Allophylus africanus*". *Chinese Journal of Natural Medicines*, 13(2):133–141.

Ola-Fadunsin, S. D. and Ademola, I. O. (2014). "Anticoccidial effects of *Morinda lucida* acetone extracts on broiler chickens naturally infected with *Eimeria* species". *Pharmaceutical Biology*, 52(3): 330–334.

Olaitan, O. J., agu, S. U., Adepoju-Bello, A. A., Nwaeze, K. U. and Olufunsho, A. (2013). "Preliminary anti-fungal activity of the aqueous bark extract of *Calotropis procera* (asclepiadaceae)". *Nigerian Quarterly Journal of Hospital Medicine*, 23(4): 338–341.

Omotoyinbo, O. V. and Sanni, M. D. (2015). "GC-MS analysis of phyto-components from the leaves of *Senna alata* L". *Journal of Plant Sciences*, 3(3): 133–136.

Oramadike, T. and Ogunbanwo, S. T. (2017). "Antagonistic activity of *:ymus vulgaris* extracts against vibrio species isolated from seafoods". *Journal of Food Science and Technology*, 54(5): 1199–1205.

Ozioma, E. O. J. and Chinwe, O. A. N. (2019). "Herbal medicines in African traditional medicine". *Herbal Medicine*, 10: 191–214.

Pavithra, P. S., Janani, V. S., Charumathi, K. H., Indumathy, R. Potala, S. and Verma, R.S. (2010). "Antibacterial activity of plants used in Indian herbal medicine". *International Journal of Green Pharmacy*, 4:22–28.

Sasidharan, S., Chen, Y., Saravanan, D., Sundram, K. M. and Latha, L. Y. (2011). "Extraction, isolation and characterization of bioactive compounds from plants' extracts". *African Journal of Traditional, Complementary and Alternative Medicines*, 8(1): 2-11.

Sheikh, A.R., Afsheen, A., Sadia, K. and Abdul, W. (2013). Plasmid borne antibiotic resistance factors among indigenous *Klebsiella. Pakistan Journal of Botany*, 35:2:243-248.

Shittu, O.B., Ajayi, O. L., Bankole, S. O. and Popoola, T. O. S. (2016)."Intestinal ameliorative effects of traditional ogi-tutu, *Vernonia amygdalina* and *Psidium guajava* in mice infected with *Vibrio cholera*". *African Health Sciences*, 16(2): 620–628.

Singh, A., Ogunbodede, E. and Onayade, A. (2013). "The role and place of medicinal plants in the strategies for disease prevention". *African Journal of Traditional, Complementary and Alternative Medicines,* 10(5): 210–229.

Singh, G., Tamboli, E., Acharya, A., Kumarasamy, C., Mala, K. and Raman, P. (2015). "Bioactive proteins from solanaceae as quorum sensing inhibitors against virulence in *Pseudomonas aeruginosa*". *Medical Hypotheses*, 84(6): 539–542.

Sofowora A. (2010). *Medicinal Plants and Traditional Medicine in Africa.* Spectrum Books Limited, Ibadan, Pp.50-195.

Suleiman, M. M., Dzenda, T. and Sani, C. A. (2018). "Antidiarrhoeal activity of the methanol stem-bark extract of *Annona senegalensis* pers. (annonaceae)". *Journal of Ethnopharmacology*, 116(1): 125–130.

Suleyman, G. and Alangaden, G. J. (2016). "Nosocomial fungal infections". *Infectious Disease Clinics of North America*, 30 (4): 1023–1052.

Taiwo, B. and Igbeneghu, O. (2014). "Antioxidant and antibacterial activities of flavonoid glycosides from ficus exasperata vahlholl (moraceae) leaves". *African Journal of Traditional, Complementary and Alternative Medicines*, 11(3): 97–101.

Tiwari, P., Kumar, B., Kaur, M., Kaur, G. and Kaur, H. (2011). "Phytochemical screening and extraction: a review". *International Journal of Pharmacy and Pharmaceutical Sciences*, 1(1): 98–106.

Udochukwu, U., Omeje, F. I., Uloma, I. S. and Oseiwe, F. D. (2015). "Phytochemical analysis of *vernonia amygdalina* and *Ocimum gratissimum* extracts and their antibacterial activity on some drug resistant bacteria". *American Journal of Respiratory and Critical Care Medicine*, 3(5): 225–235.

Ugboko, H., Mathew, B., Solomon, R., Omonigbehin, E. and De, N. (2016). "Studies on effects of bark extracts of *Azadirachta indica* a. (juss) on multidrug resistant *Salmonella typhi*". *Asian Journal of Applied Science and Technology*, 7(2): 2325–2332.

Ukamaka, O., Paul, N. and Ikechi, E. (2015). "Antiviral effects of *Nauclea latifolia* on newcastle disease virus (NDV)". *Sky Journal of Microbiology Research*, 3: 1–5.

Uzodimma, D. E. (2013). "Medico-ethnobotanical inventory of ogii, okigwe imostate, south eastern Nigeria". *Global Journal of Medicinal Plants Research*, 2(2):30–44.

Vambe, M., Aremu, A. O., Chukwujekwu, J.C., Finnie, J. F. and Van Staden, J. (2018). "Antibacterial screening, synergy studies and phenolic content of seven south African medicinal plants against drug-sensitive and resistant microbial strains". *South African Journal of Botany*, 114: 250–259.

World Health Organization (WHO). (2010). "Regulatory Situation of Herbal Medicine: A World Wide Review".

YOUR KNOWLEDGE HAS VALUE

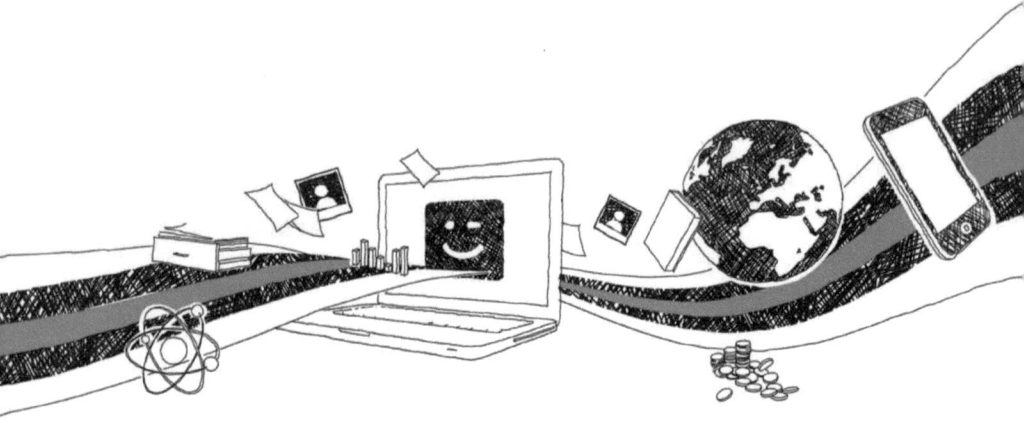

- We will publish your bachelor's and
  master's thesis, essays and papers

- Your own eBook and book -
  sold worldwide in all relevant shops

- Earn money with each sale

Upload your text at www.GRIN.com
and publish for free

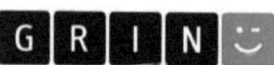